VEGAN DIET FOR RADIANT SKIN

Savoring Plant Elixirs: Unveiling Skin's Inner Glow

GLEN N. QUIRK

© [2023] [GLEN N. QUIRK]

All rights reserved. No part of this publication may be reproduced, stored in a retrieval system, or transmitted in any form or by any means, electronic, mechanical, photocopying, recording, or otherwise, without the prior written permission of the publisher.

Table of content

Introduction...................................... 7

Why Radiant Skin Matters: 9

The Power of a Vegan Lifestyle: 11

Chapter 1: The Skin-Deep Connection................................13

Recognizing the Connection Between Nutrition and Skin Health.. 13

Common Skin Issues and Their Root Causes:.. 15

Acne:.. 15

Eczema:.. 15

Psoriasis: 16

Premature Aging: 16

How a Plant-Based Diet Can Change Your Skin: 16

Nutrient Density of Plant-Based Foods:....... 16

ated.

Chapter 2: Nutrient-Rich Foundations 19

Essential Nutrients for Healthy Skin: 19

Antioxidants: The Skin's Natural Defenses: 21

The Fatty Acids Omega-3: Eating Healthily from the Inside Out: 23

Minerals and Vitamins: The Components That Make Up Radiance 25

Chapter 3: Plant-Powered Glow 27

Revealing the Magnificence of Vegetarian Diets: 27

The Rainbow Plate: Consuming Vibrant Foods 29

Super foods to Boost Skin Power: 31

Chapter 4: Crafting Your Radiant Menu....................... 33

Sample Meal Plans: 33

Day 1: 33

Day 2: 33

Day 3: 33

Day 4: 34

Day 5: 34

Day 6 34

Day 7: 34

Day 8: 35

Day 9: 35

Day 10: 35

Day 11: 35

Day 12: 36

Day 13: 36

Day 14: 36

Breakfasts to Kick start Your Day 36

Lunches for Sustained Energy 54

Delicious Dinners for Skin Renewal 73

Snacks recipes 84

Dessert recipes 99

Healthy fruit to include................................... 116

Tips for Radiant Skin: 121

Chapter 5: Transitioning from the Kitchen to the Vanity 123

DIY Beauty Treatments: Harnessing the Power of Plants 123

Homemade Masks for Radiant Skin: 123

Natural Cleansers and Toners: 125

Plant-Powered Moisturizers:......................... 126

Chapter 6: Beyond the Plate 129

The Comprehensive Guide to Radiant Skin through a Holistic Approach........................ 129

Conclusion 133

INTRODUCTION

Mary's journey to radiant health started with a simple decision to adopt a vegan lifestyle. Driven by a desire for holistic well-being, her decision to follow a vegan diet unfolded like the opening chapter of a compelling novel. In the midst of a fast-paced, bustling city, Mary found herself yearning for something more. Her skin, which had previously been dull and prone to breakouts, was a reflection of the stress and imbalance in her life. Determining to restore her vitality, Mary set out to find a solution that went beyond traditional skincare routines.

When Mary learned about the transformational potential of a vegan diet, it was a game-changer. She researched plant-based nutrition, drawn by its claims to nurture her body from the inside out. Mary learned that having beautiful skin has more to do with her kitchen decisions than merely applying topical treatments.

Mary started to see changes in her skin as she embraced the rainbow of fruits, veggies, and whole grains. Her inner light began to serve as a daily reminder that she was headed in the correct direction. With every satisfying plant-based meal, Mary fed her body and her newly discovered life passion.

The story developed as Mary played around with inventive vegan meals, creating a menu that not only pleased her palate but also provided her skin with much-needed nutrition. Mary's kitchen transformed into a haven for skin-loving ingredients, serving everything from delectable plant-based dinners to nutrient-dense smoothie bowls for breakfast.

Nobody missed her brilliant metamorphosis. Mary's friends and coworkers were astounded by her renewed vigor and wanted to know her secret. Mary talked about how following a vegan diet has helped her achieve glowing health while smiling.

What started off as a personal search for colorful skin turned into an inspirational tale. Mary's brilliant glow attracted others to the plant-based lifestyle by acting as a beacon. By skillfully navigating social situations and dispelling common misconceptions about veganism, Mary unintentionally became a spokesperson for a way of life that went beyond the plate.

The pages of Mary's story turned not only with the passage of time but also with each satisfying meal, every kind word, and every person she motivated. The beginning of Mary's story serves as an introduction to a story that goes beyond nutrition; it's a journey of self-awareness, wellbeing, and the radiant metamorphosis that happens when a woman decides to use the power of a vegan lifestyle to nurture her body and spirit.

Why Radiant Skin Matters:

Radiant skin is not merely a superficial aesthetic; it serves as a mirror reflecting our overall health and well-being. The skin is the body's largest organ, and its condition often reveals much about our internal state. Beyond societal standards of beauty, radiant skin signifies vitality, balance, and a harmonious relationship with our environment.

When our skin is healthy, it functions as a protective barrier, shielding us from external pollutants, UV rays, and harmful microbes. A radiant complexion often suggests optimal hydration, proper nutrition, and efficient detoxification processes within the body. Moreover, the confidence that comes with healthy, glowing skin can positively impact our mental and emotional well-being.

Conversely, skin conditions may serve as markers for underlying medical conditions. Inflammation, dullness, and acne can all be indicators of toxic exposure, dietary imbalances, or stress. Understanding the importance of glowing skin inspires us to take a holistic approach to health, taking into account both topical therapies and treating the underlying causes of skin issues.

Radiant skin is important because it basically shows the balance of our body's internal systems, gives an indication of our general health, and boosts our confidence and sense of self-worth in the way we show ourselves to the outside world.

The Power of a Vegan Lifestyle:

Beyond only changing one's diet, adopting a vegan lifestyle involves a significant shift toward compassionate living and holistic wellbeing. Adopting a vegan diet enables people to make ethical judgments about the treatment of animals and the environment, as well as considerations that go well beyond their own health.

A vegan diet involves eating a lot of plant-based foods that are high in vitamins, minerals, antioxidants, fiber, and other nutrients. These components are essential for maintaining proper organ function, enhancing general well-being, and, most importantly, improving skin health and vibrancy.

Because plant-based nutrition has many intrinsic benefits, leading a vegan lifestyle can be an effective weapon in the quest for glowing skin. A wide range of nutrients found in fruits, vegetables, nuts, seeds, and legumes hydrate the skin from the inside out while encouraging the production of collagen and fending against oxidative stress.

Furthermore, a vegan lifestyle has an even greater impact because to its ethical and environmental aspects. People may lessen their carbon footprint, mitigate deforestation, and advance a more sustainable, cruelty-free society by making plant-based dietary choices.

To sum up, the efficacy of a vegan diet is rooted in its capacity to advance personal well-being, augment skin brightness, and expand its beneficial impact into the wider realm of ethical and environmental concerns. It's a decision that has a profound impact on one's personal health as well as the health of the world and all of its inhabitants.

CHAPTER 1: THE SKIN-DEEP CONNECTION

Recognizing the Connection Between Nutrition and Skin Health

The connection between diet and skin health is a complex interplay that goes beyond surface-level beauty. The skin, being the body's largest organ, is profoundly influenced by the nutrients we consume. Understanding this link involves acknowledging the impact of various dietary elements on the skin's structure, function, and overall appearance.

Nutrient Deficiencies and Skin Health:

Essential nutrients, such as vitamins A, C, and E, as well as minerals like zinc, contribute to skin health. Deficiencies in these nutrients can lead to issues like dryness, premature aging, and a compromised ability to repair and regenerate.

Inflammation and Skin Conditions:

Certain dietary choices, like consuming processed foods, excessive sugars, and unhealthy fats, can contribute to systemic inflammation. Chronic inflammation is linked to skin conditions such as acne, psoriasis, and eczema.

Hydration and Skin Elasticity:

Adequate hydration is fundamental for maintaining skin elasticity and preventing dryness. Dehydration can make the skin more prone to fine lines and wrinkles, emphasizing the importance of consuming enough water and water-rich foods.

Gut Health and Skin Conditions:

The relationship between intestinal health and skin disorders is highlighted by the gut-skin axis. A diet rich in fiber and probiotics supports a healthy gut micro biome, potentially reducing inflammation and improving skin conditions.

Understanding the link between diet and skin health involves recognizing how the foods we eat influence not only the external appearance of the skin but also its internal processes and ability to function as a protective barrier.

Common Skin Issues and Their Root Causes:

Acne:

Root Causes: Hormonal fluctuations, excess sebum production, inflammation, and a diet high in processed foods and dairy can contribute to the development of acne.

Eczema:

Root Causes: Genetic predisposition, immune system dysfunction, environmental factors, and dietary triggers such as gluten and dairy can play a role in the development and exacerbation of eczema.

Psoriasis:

Root Causes: Genetic factors, immune system over activity, stress, and dietary factors like alcohol and red meat may contribute to the development and exacerbation of psoriasis.

Premature Aging:

Root Causes: Exposure to UV rays, environmental pollutants, smoking, and a diet lacking in antioxidants can accelerate the aging process, leading to wrinkles, fine lines, and sagging skin.

How a Plant-Based Diet Can Change Your Skin:

Nutrient Density of Plant-Based Foods:

A vegan diet, rich in fruits, vegetables, nuts, seeds, and whole grains, provides a broad spectrum of essential nutrients. These include vitamins, minerals, and antioxidants crucial for skin health, supporting collagen production and protecting against oxidative stress.

Anti-Inflammatory Properties:

Plant-based diets are known for their anti-inflammatory properties, helping to mitigate inflammation associated with various skin conditions. Reduction in inflammation can lead to clearer skin and a more even complexion.

Hydration from Plant Foods:

Fruits and vegetables, among other plant-based foods, are high in water content. This contributes to internal hydration, promoting plump and supple skin. Proper hydration is vital for maintaining the skin's moisture barrier.

Balancing Hormones:

Hormonal imbalances can contribute to skin issues, especially acne. Plant-based diets, with their potential to regulate hormonal levels, may lead to improvements in hormonal acne and other related conditions.

Reducing Environmental Impact:

A vegan diet aligns with environmental sustainability, reducing the ecological footprint associated with animal agriculture. A healthier planet indirectly contributes to a healthier environment for your skin.

The understanding of the link between diet and skin health reveals a dynamic relationship where the choices we make at the dining table have far-reaching effects on the health and appearance of our skin. Embracing a vegan diet can be a transformative step toward nurturing your skin from the inside out, promoting not only external radiance but also overall well-being.

Chapter 2: Nutrient-Rich Foundations

Essential Nutrients for Healthy Skin:

A sufficient intake of vital nutrients is necessary to attain and preserve healthy skin, as these nutrients are vital to the construction, function, and general health of the skin.

Proteins:

Proteins are necessary for the regeneration and repair of skin. Structure and suppleness are imparted by collagen, a protein that is prevalent in the skin. Skin health is supported by a diet high in protein sources including quinoa, lentils, tofu, and beans.

Water:

Skin hydration and suppleness are fundamentally dependent on it. Water facilitates the removal of pollutants and the delivery of nutrients to skin cells. To keep skin hydrated, one must consume enough water and meals high in water.

Essential Fatty Acids:

Omega-3 and omega-6 essential fatty acids are particularly important for the health of the skin. They aid in the development of a strong skin barrier, which stops moisture loss. Walnuts, hemp seeds, chia seeds, flaxseeds, and walnut oil are sources of omega-3 fatty acids.

Vitamins (A, C, and E):

In order to promote a healthy complexion, vitamin A supports sebum production and skin cell turnover. In addition to being an antioxidant that shields the skin from oxidative damage, vitamin C is necessary for the creation of collagen. Another antioxidant that supports skin preservation and hydration is vitamin E.

Minerals (selenium, zinc):

Selenium supports antioxidant defense, whereas zinc aids in skin cell renewal and repair. Both minerals have an effect in shielding the skin from harm from the environment. Good sources of zinc and selenium include nuts, seeds, whole grains, and legumes.

Biotin:

B-vitamin biotin promotes skin cell health and may help avoid dry skin. Foods include spinach, sweet potatoes, almonds, and seeds contain it.

Antioxidants: The Skin's Natural Defenses:

Strong substances called antioxidants scavenge free radicals, avoiding oxidative stress and cell damage, including skin damage. Bright, protected skin can be achieved by include a range of foods high in antioxidants in your diet.

Vitamin C:

Vitamin C, a strong antioxidant that supports collagen synthesis, guards against UV damage, and evens out skin tone, is found in citrus fruits, berries, and leafy greens.

Vitamin E:

Vegetable oils, seeds, and nuts are rich sources of vitamin E. This antioxidant maintains the general health of the skin while shielding it from environmental damage.

Beta-carotene:

Found in orange and yellow produce such as sweet potatoes, carrots, and mangoes, beta-carotene is transformed into vitamin A to help protect and repair skin.

Flavonoids:

Flavonoids, which are present in tea, fruits, and vegetables, have anti-inflammatory and antioxidant qualities that assist to protect skin from oxidative stress.

Polyphenols:

Polyphenols, which are abundant in berries, dark chocolate, and green tea, help hydrate the skin and shield it from UV rays.

The Fatty Acids Omega-3: Eating Healthily from the Inside Out:

Essential fats that the body is unable to create on its own are omega-3 fatty acids. They offer several advantages for general well-being and are essential for preserving the health of the skin.

ALA, or alpha-linolenic acid,

ALA, an omega-3 fatty acid derived from plants, is present in walnuts, chia seeds, and flaxseeds. It helps maintain the hydration and flexibility of the skin.

The compounds docosahexaenoic acid (DHA) and eicosapentaenoic acid (EPA):

The fatty acids EPA and DHA, which are frequently present in salmon and mackerel, help to moisturize and reduce inflammation in the skin.

Cut Down on Inflammation:

Omega-3 fatty acids assist in reducing the body's inflammatory reactions, which are linked to diseases like psoriasis, eczema, and acne.

Counteracting UV Damage:

According to certain research, omega-3 fatty acids may assist in shielding the skin from UV radiation's damaging effects and lowering the chance of sun damage.

Minerals and Vitamins: The Components That Make Up Radiance:

The fundamental components of glowing skin are vitamins and minerals, which are essential to many physiological functions that affect the condition and look of the skin.

Vitamin A

Vitamin A helps prevent diseases like acne and supports a healthy complexion by being essential for skin cell turnover and repair. Carrots, sweet potatoes, and leafy greens are some examples of sources.

Vitamin C

Vitamin C is essential for the production of collagen and enhances the suppleness and toughness of skin. Citrus fruits, bell peppers, and strawberries are excellent sources.

Vitamin E

Almonds, sunflower seeds, and spinach are good
sources of vitamin E, an antioxidant that guards
against oxidative damage to skin cells.

Zinc

helps regulate the production of oil and promotes
the renewal and repair of skin cells. Zinc-rich foods
include lentils, chickpeas, and pumpkin seeds.

Selenium

Selenium is a trace mineral that functions as an
antioxidant and shields the skin from harm from the
environment. Whole grains, sunflower seeds, and
brazil nuts are excellent sources.

vitamins B: riboflavin, niacin, and biotin

Niacin aids in skin hydration, biotin promotes
healthy skin, and riboflavin assists the preservation
of skin structure. Many foods, such as nuts, seeds,
whole grains, and leafy greens, contain these
vitamins.

Including a variety of foods high in nutrients in
your diet guarantees that your skin will get the
nutrients it needs to be as healthy and radiant as
possible.

Chapter 3: Plant-Powered Glow

Revealing the Magnificence of Vegetarian Diets:

In addition to being a dietary decision, adopting a plant-based lifestyle involves exploring the wide and colorful world of plant-based foods, each of which has special advantages for your overall health and wellbeing. Plant-based foods are the cornerstone of a diet that nourishes your body from the inside out. These foods range from nutrient-rich veggies to protein-packed legumes and entire grains.

Nutrient Diversity:

Full of vitamins, minerals, antioxidants, and fiber, plant-based diets are a great source of vital nutrients. This wide-ranging nutritional profile promotes general health, increases vitality, and leaves your skin looking gorgeous.

Enhancing Digestive Health:

The high fiber content of plant-based diets supports a balanced gut microbiota. Your skin's health and look can be enhanced by effective digestion and nutrient absorption, both of which are facilitated by a gut that is in balance.

Properties that Reduce Inflammation:

Anti-inflammatory qualities found in a wide variety of plant-based foods aid in the body's reduction of inflammation. Numerous skin disorders are associated with chronic inflammation, and a plant-based diet may be a natural means of reducing this problem.

Plant-Based Hydration:

Because fruits and vegetables are high in water, they help keep the body hydrated on the surface as well as within cells. Sustaining a healthy complexion and preserving skin hydration depend on proper hydration.

Sustainability of the Environment:

Eating a plant-based diet contributes to environmental sustainability since it lowers the carbon footprint of animal agriculture. A healthier Earth benefits everyone and everything on it, including your skin, in addition to the ecosystem.

The Rainbow Plate: Consuming Vibrant Foods

A "rainbow plate" is made up of a variety of vibrant fruits and vegetables, each of which represents a different set of phytonutrients and health advantages.

Red:

Antioxidants with anti-aging and anti-inflammatory qualities, such as lycopene and anthocyanins, are abundant in tomatoes, red peppers, and berries.

Yellow and Orange:

Beta-carotene, which is believed to promote a vibrant complexion and is crucial for skin health, may be found in carrots, sweet potatoes, oranges, and mangoes.

Green:

Broccoli, kiwi, and leafy greens are rich in minerals, vitamins, and chlorophyll, which promote the creation of collagen and the general health of the skin.

Purple and Blue:

Antioxidants called anthocyanins are found in eggplants, blackberries, and blueberries. They may help shield the skin from oxidative stress and give it a more youthful appearance.

Brown and White:

Whole grains, mushrooms, and cauliflower are good sources of selenium and other minerals that support the health and vigor of the skin.

Placing a diverse range of plant-based foods on your plate guarantees a wide range of nutrients, which supports general wellbeing as well as skin health.

Super foods to Boost Skin Power:

Some plant-based foods are considered "super foods" because of their high nutrient density and possible advantages for skin health.

Berries:

Antioxidants found in blueberries, strawberries, and raspberries shield the skin from damage caused by free radicals and help to maintain a youthful complexion.

Avocado:

Avocado supports skin hydration and suppleness since it is a rich source of biotin, vitamin E, and healthy monounsaturated fats.

Greens with leaves:

Powerhouse greens like kale, spinach, and Swiss chard are high in vitamins A, C, and K, which promote the creation of collagen and general skin health.

Chia Seeds:

Omega-3 fatty acids, which are found in chia seeds, help hydrate the skin and lower inflammation.

Turmeric

Curcumin, an antioxidant and anti-inflammatory compound found in turmeric, may help treat skin disorders like psoriasis and acne.

Walnuts:

Omega-3 fatty acids and vitamin E found in walnuts promote skin suppleness and guard against oxidative damage.

Tomatoes:

Lycopene, which is abundant in tomatoes, protects the skin from UV rays and promotes healthy skin.

By including these superfoods in your plant-based diet, you may improve the nutrition your skin gets and look younger and healthier. To achieve the best skin advantages, always remember that the secret is to embrace variety and indulge in a wide variety of plant-based diets.

Chapter 4: Crafting Your Radiant Menu

Sample Meal Plans:

Day 1:

Breakfast: Berry Smoothie Bowl

Lunch: Vegan Mediterranean Wrap

Dinner: Stuffed Bell Peppers

Day 2:

Breakfast: Avocado Toast with Tomatoes

Lunch: Lentil and Vegetable Curry

Dinner: Zucchini Noodles with Pesto

Day 3:

Breakfast: Quinoa Breakfast Bowl

Lunch: Mushroom and Spinach Stuffed Bell Peppers

Dinner: Vegan Sushi Bowl

Breakfast: Vegan Oatmeal with Berries

Lunch: Quinoa and Vegetable Stir-Fry

Dinner: Vegan Caesar Salad

Breakfast: Chia Seed Pudding

Lunch: Chickpea and Spinach Curry

Dinner: Tomato Basil Zucchini Noodles

Breakfast: Kale and Chickpea Salad

Lunch: Sweet Potato and Lentil Soup

Dinner: Butternut Squash and Lentil Stew

Breakfast: Almond Butter and Banana Slices

Lunch: Vegan Blueberry Pancakes

Dinner: Coconut Mango Sorbet

Breakfast: Carrot Sticks with Hummus

Lunch: Acai Bowl with Granola

Dinner: Vegan Berry Tart

Breakfast: Mixed Berry Parfait

Lunch: Chocolate Peanut Butter Overnight Oats

Dinner: Vegan Mediterranean Bowl

Breakfast: Kale Chips

Lunch: Energy Bites

Dinner: Stuffed Dates

Breakfast: Avocado Chocolate Mousse

Lunch: Vegan Breakfast Burrito

Dinner: Pineapple Coconut Nice Cream

Breakfast: Chia Seed Pudding Parfait

Lunch: Roasted Chickpeas

Dinner: Homemade Trail Mix

Breakfast: Frozen Banana Ice Cream

Lunch: Veggie Sticks with Guacamole

Dinner: Almond Joy Energy Balls

Breakfast: Mango Coconut Rice Pudding

Lunch: Berry Chia Seed Jam

Dinner: Banana Walnut Bread

Breakfasts to Kick start Your Day

Berry Smoothie Bowl:

Ingredients:

1 cup mixed berries (strawberries, blueberries, raspberries)

1 banana

1/2 cup spinach leaves

1/2 cup almond milk

1 tablespoon chia seeds

Toppings: Granola, sliced strawberries, chia seeds, coconut flakes

Preparation Method:

Combine mixed berries, banana, spinach, and almond milk in a blender.

Blend until smooth and creamy.

Pour the smoothie into a bowl.

Sprinkle granola, chia seeds, coconut flakes, and sliced strawberries on top.

Instructions:

Customize toppings based on preference.

Experiment with different berries for variety.

Cooking Time: 5 minutes

Total Making Time: 10 minutes

Serving Size: 1

Nutrition Value:

Calories: 350

Protein: 8g

Fiber: 12g

Vitamin C: 90mg

Iron: 3mg

Avocado Toast with Tomatoes:

Ingredients:

1 slice whole-grain bread

1/2 ripe avocado

Cherry tomatoes, sliced

Salt and pepper to taste

Red pepper flakes (optional)

Fresh cilantro or basil for garnish

Preparation Method:

Toast the whole-grain bread slice.

Spread the mashed, ripe avocado over the toast.

Top with sliced cherry tomatoes.

Add salt, pepper, and red pepper flakes for seasoning, if preferred.

Garnish with fresh cilantro or basil.

Instructions:

Drizzle with a touch of olive oil for added flavor.

Cooking Time: 5 minutes

Total Making Time: 10 minutes

Serving Size: 1

Nutrition Value:

Calories: 220

Healthy Fats: 15g

Fiber: 8g

Vitamin C: 15mg

Potassium: 550mg

Chia Seed Pudding:

Ingredients:

3 tablespoons chia seeds

1 cup almond milk

1/2 teaspoon vanilla extract

Fresh berries for topping

Maple syrup for sweetness (optional)

Preparation Method:

Combine chia seeds, almond milk, and vanilla essence in a bowl.

Stir well and let it sit for 5 minutes.

Stir again, cover, and refrigerate overnight.

In the morning, give it a final stir and top with fresh berries.

Optionally, drizzle with maple syrup for sweetness.

Instructions:

Customize with your favorite fruits and nuts.

Cooking Time: 5 minutes (plus overnight refrigeration)

Total Making Time: 8 hours

Serving Size: 1

Nutrition Value:

Calories: 220

Omega-3 Fatty Acids: 5g

Fiber: 16g

Protein: 6g

Calcium: 300mg

Quinoa Breakfast Bowl:

Ingredients:

1/2 cup cooked quinoa

1/2 cup almond milk

1 tablespoon almond butter

Sliced banana

Chopped nuts (walnuts or almonds)

Dried fruits (raisins or cranberries)

Cinnamon for flavor

Preparation Method:

Almond milk and cooked quinoa should be combined in a bowl.

Stir in almond butter and mix well.

Add chopped nuts, dried fruits, and sliced banana on top.

Sprinkle with cinnamon for added flavor.

Instructions:

Adjust sweetness by adding a drizzle of maple syrup if desired.

Cooking Time: 15 minutes (for pre-cooked quinoa)

Total Making Time: 20 minutes

Serving Size: 1

Nutrition Value:

Calories: 350

Protein: 9g

Fiber: 8g

Healthy Fats: 15g

Iron: 2mg

Vegan Oatmeal with Berries:

Ingredients:

1/2 cup rolled oats

1 cup almond milk

Mixed berries (strawberries, blueberries, raspberries)

1 tablespoon maple syrup

Chopped nuts (almonds or walnuts)

Cinnamon for flavor

Preparation Method:

Almond milk and rolled oats should be combined in a saucepan.

Cook until creamy, stirring periodically, over medium heat for the oats.

Top with mixed berries, maple syrup, and chopped nuts.

Sprinkle with cinnamon for added flavor.

Instructions:

Experiment with different berry combinations.

Cooking Time: 10 minutes

Total Making Time: 15 minutes

Serving Size: 1

Nutrition Value:

Calories: 300

Protein: 8g

Fiber: 10g

Vitamin C: 30mg

Calcium: 200mg

Vegan Blueberry Pancakes:

Ingredients:

1 cup whole wheat flour

1 tablespoon baking powder

1 tablespoon sugar

1 cup almond milk

1/2 cup fresh blueberries

Coconut oil for cooking

Preparation Method:

In a bowl, whisk together flour, baking powder, and sugar.

Gradually add almond milk, stirring to form a smooth batter.

Gently fold in fresh blueberries.

Heat a skillet with coconut oil and spoon batter for each pancake.

Stir and continue cooking until bubbles form and the food turns golden brown.

Instructions:

Serve with additional blueberries and a drizzle of maple syrup.

Cooking Time: 15 minutes

Total Making Time: 25 minutes

Serving Size: 2-3

Nutrition Value:

Calories: 220 (per pancake)

Protein: 6g

Fiber: 4g

Vitamin C: 8mg

Iron: 1mg

Green Smoothie with Spirulina:

Ingredients:

1 cup spinach leaves

1/2 banana

1/2 cup pineapple chunks

1/2 cup coconut water

1 teaspoon spirulina powder

Ice cubes for a chilled smoothie

Preparation Method:

Combine spinach, banana, pineapple, coconut water, and spirulina in a blender.

Blend until smooth and creamy.

Add ice cubes and blend again for a chilled smoothie.

Instructions:

Adjust sweetness by adding more banana or a touch of honey.

Cooking Time: 5 minutes

Total Making Time: 10 minutes

Serving Size: 1

Nutrition Value:

Calories: 150

Protein: 3g

Fiber: 4g

Vitamin A: 1500 IU

Iron: 2mg

Chocolate Peanut Butter Overnight Oats:

Ingredients:

1/2 cup rolled oats

1/2 cup almond milk

1 tablespoon cocoa powder

1 tablespoon peanut butter

Sliced banana for topping

Chopped nuts for topping

Preparation Method:

In a jar, combine rolled oats, almond milk, cocoa powder, and peanut butter.

Stir well and refrigerate overnight.

In the morning, top with sliced banana and chopped nuts.

Instructions:

For added taste, drizzle some more peanut butter over it.

Cooking Time: 5 minutes (plus overnight refrigeration)

Total Making Time: 8 hours

Serving Size: 1

Nutrition Value:

Calories: 350

Protein: 9g

Fiber: 8g

Healthy Fats: 15g

Iron: 2mg

Vegan Breakfast Burrito:

Ingredients:

1 whole-grain wrap

1/2 cup tofu scramble

1/4 cup black beans, cooked

Salsa for topping

Avocado slices for topping

Fresh cilantro for garnish

Preparation Method:

Warm the whole-grain wrap.

Fill the wrap with tofu scramble and black beans.

Top with salsa and avocado slices.

Garnish with fresh cilantro.

Instructions:

Add a dash of hot sauce for extra spice.

Cooking Time: 10 minutes

Total Making Time: 15 minutes

Serving Size: 1

Nutrition Value:

Calories: 300

Protein: 15g

Fiber: 8g

Healthy Fats: 10g

Iron: 2mg

Acai Bowl with Granola:

Ingredients:

Acai puree packet

1/2 cup mixed berries

1/4 cup granola

Sliced banana for topping

Chia seeds for topping

Drizzle of honey for sweetness (optional)

Preparation Method:

Blend the acai puree packet with mixed berries until smooth.

Pour the acai blend into a bowl.

Top with granola, sliced banana, and chia seeds.

Optionally, drizzle with honey for sweetness.

Instructions:

Experiment with different toppings like shredded coconut or nuts.

Cooking Time: 5 minutes

Total Making Time: 10 minutes

Serving Size: 1

Nutrition Value:

Calories: 250

Protein: 5g

Fiber: 6g

Antioxidants: 5000 IU

Calcium: 100mg

Lunches for Sustained Energy

Kale and Chickpea Salad:

Ingredients:

Kale leaves, stems removed

Chickpeas, cooked

Cherry tomatoes, halved

Cucumber, sliced

Red onion, thinly sliced

Avocado, diced

Lemon-tahini dressing

Preparation Method:

To soften, massage some olive oil into the kale leaves.

In a large bowl, combine kale, chickpeas, cherry tomatoes, cucumber, red onion, and avocado.

Drizzle with lemon-tahini dressing and toss until well coated.

Instructions:

Toss the salad just before serving for the best texture.

Cooking Time: None (No cooking involved)

Total Making Time: 15 minutes

Serving Size: 2

Nutrition Value:

Calories: 350

Protein: 15g

Fiber: 12g

Healthy Fats: 18g

Quinoa and Vegetable Stir-Fry:

Ingredients:

Quinoa, cooked

Mixed vegetables (bell peppers, broccoli, carrots)

Tofu, cubed

Soy sauce

Sesame oil

Garlic, minced

Ginger, grated

Preparation Method:

In a pan, stir-fry tofu until golden brown. Set aside.

In the same pan, sauté garlic and ginger. Add mixed vegetables and stir-fry until tender.

Add cooked quinoa and tofu to the vegetables.

Drizzle with soy sauce and sesame oil. Toss until well combined.

Instructions:

Adjust soy sauce and sesame oil to taste.

Cooking Time: 20 minutes

Total Making Time: 30 minutes

Serving Size: 4

Nutrition Value:

Calories: 300

Protein: 14g

Fiber: 8g

Healthy Fats: 10g

Sweet Potato and Lentil Soup:

Ingredients:

Sweet potatoes, peeled and diced

Red lentils, rinsed

Onion, chopped

Garlic, minced

Vegetable broth

Coconut milk

Curry powder

Turmeric

Salt and pepper, to taste

Preparation Method:

Fry the garlic and onion in a pot until they become tender.

Add sweet potatoes, red lentils, curry powder, turmeric, salt, and pepper.

After adding the veggie broth, bring it to a boil. Simmer until sweet potatoes and lentils are tender.

Blend the soup until smooth. Stir in coconut milk.

Instructions:

Adjust seasonings to taste.

Cooking Time: 30 minutes

Total Making Time: 45 minutes

Serving Size: 6

Nutrition Value:

Calories: 220

Protein: 8g

Fiber: 10g

Healthy Fats: 5g

Cauliflower and Broccoli Bowl:

Ingredients:

Cauliflower, florets

Broccoli, florets

Quinoa, cooked

Almonds, sliced

Lemon-tahini dressing

Preparation Method:

Steam cauliflower and broccoli until tender.

In a bowl, combine steamed vegetables with cooked quinoa.

Drizzle with lemon-tahini dressing and top with sliced almonds.

Instructions:

Garnish with fresh herbs if desired.

Cooking Time: 15 minutes

Total Making Time: 25 minutes

Serving Size: 3

Nutrition Value:

Calories: 280

Protein: 12g

Fiber: 9g

Healthy Fats: 8g

Vegan Mediterranean Wrap:

Ingredients:

Whole-grain wraps

Hummus

Falafel

Cucumber, sliced

Tomato, diced

Red onion, thinly sliced

Kalamata olives, sliced

Fresh parsley, chopped

Preparation Method:

Spread hummus on the wraps.

Add falafel, cucumber, tomato, red onion, olives, and parsley.

Roll the wraps tightly.

Instructions:

Serve immediately or wrap in parchment paper for later.

Cooking Time: 20 minutes (if making falafel from scratch)

Total Making Time: 30 minutes

Serving Size: 2

Nutrition Value:

Calories: 380

Protein: 15g

Fiber: 10g

Healthy Fats: 12g

Mushroom and Spinach Stuffed Bell Peppers:

Ingredients:

Bell peppers, halved

Mushrooms, chopped

Spinach, chopped

Quinoa, cooked

Garlic, minced

Tomato sauce

Italian seasoning

Vegan cheese, grated

Preparation Method:

Preheat the oven. Bell peppers should be put in a baking dish.

In a skillet, sauté mushrooms, spinach, and garlic until wilted.

Stir in cooked quinoa, tomato sauce, and Italian seasoning.

Stuff bell peppers with the quinoa mixture. Top with vegan cheese.

Bake until peppers are tender.

Instructions:

Garnish with fresh herbs before serving.

Cooking Time: 30 minutes

Total Making Time: 50 minutes

Serving Size: 4

Nutrition Value:

Calories: 250

Protein: 10g

Fiber: 8g

Healthy Fats: 7g

Vegan Mediterranean Bowl:

Ingredients:

Quinoa, cooked

Chickpeas, cooked

Cherry tomatoes, halved

Cucumber, diced

Red onion, finely chopped

Kalamata olives, sliced

Hummus

Lemon-tahini dressing

Preparation Method:

In a bowl, arrange quinoa, chickpeas, cherry tomatoes, cucumber, red onion, and olives.

Drizzle with hummus and lemon-tahini dressing.

Instructions:

Mix well before eating.

Cooking Time: 20 minutes

Total Making Time: 30 minutes

Serving Size: 3

Nutrition Value:

Calories: 320

Protein: 12g

Fiber: 9g

Healthy Fats: 10g

Chickpea and Spinach Curry:

Ingredients:

Chickpeas, cooked

Spinach, chopped

Coconut milk

Onion, finely chopped

Garlic, minced

Ginger, grated

Curry spices (turmeric, cumin, coriander)

Tomato, diced

Preparation Method:

Sauté onion, garlic, and ginger until softened.

Add curry spices and cook until fragrant.

Stir in chickpeas, spinach, coconut milk, and diced
tomatoes.

Simmer until the spinach wilts.

Instructions:

Serve over rice or quinoa.

Cooking Time: 25 minutes

Total Making Time: 40 minutes

Serving Size: 4

Nutrition Value:

Calories: 280

Protein: 11g

Fiber: 8g

Healthy Fats: 9g

Tomato Basil Zucchini Noodles:

Ingredients:

Zucchini noodles

Cherry tomatoes, halved

Garlic, minced

Fresh basil, chopped

Olive oil

Lemon juice

Pine nuts (optional)

Preparation Method:

In a pan, sauté garlic in olive oil until fragrant.

Add zucchini noodles and cherry tomatoes. Cook until just tender.

Toss with fresh basil and lemon juice.

Top with pine nuts if desired.

Instructions:

Garnish with extra basil before serving.

Cooking Time: 15 minutes

Total Making Time: 25 minutes

Serving Size: 2

Nutrition Value:

Calories: 180

Protein: 5g

Fiber: 4g

Healthy Fats: 10g

Vegan Caesar Salad:

Ingredients:

Romaine lettuce, chopped

Croutons

Vegan Caesar dressing

Cherry tomatoes, halved

Vegan Parmesan cheese, grated

Preparation Method:

In a large bowl, combine chopped romaine lettuce, croutons, and cherry tomatoes.

Toss with vegan Caesar dressing.

Sprinkle vegan Parmesan cheese on top.

Instructions:

Serve immediately for the best texture.

Cooking Time: None (No cooking involved)

Total Making Time: 15 minutes

Serving Size: 2

Nutrition Value:

Calories: 250

Protein: 7g

Fiber: 5g

Healthy Fats: 8g

Butternut Squash and Lentil Stew:

Ingredients:

Butternut squash, peeled and diced

Red lentils, rinsed

Onion, chopped

Garlic, minced

Vegetable broth

Coconut milk

Curry powder

Turmeric

Salt and pepper, to taste

Preparation Method:

Fry the garlic and onion in a pot until they become tender.

Add butternut squash, red lentils, curry powder, turmeric, salt, and pepper.

Add the vegetable broth and heat until it boils. Simmer until squash and lentils are tender.

Stir in coconut milk.

Instructions:

Adjust seasonings to taste.

Cooking Time: 30 minutes

Total Making Time: 45 minutes

Serving Size: 6

Nutrition Value:

Calories: 230

Protein: 9g

Fiber: 8g

Healthy Fats: 6g

Delicious Dinners for Skin Renewal

Stuffed Bell Peppers:

Ingredients:

Cut in half and seeded four large bell peppers

1 cup quinoa, cooked

One can (15 oz) of rinsed and drained black beans

1 cup corn kernels (fresh or frozen)

1 cup cherry tomatoes, diced

1 cup red onion, finely chopped

1 cup spinach, chopped

1 teaspoon cumin

1 teaspoon chili powder

Salt and pepper to taste

1 cup tomato sauce

1 cup vegan cheese, shredded (optional)

Preparation Method:

Preheat the oven to 375°F (190°C).

In a large mixing bowl, combine cooked quinoa, black beans, corn, cherry tomatoes, red onion, spinach, cumin, chili powder, salt, and pepper.

Stuff the quinoa mixture into each side of a bell pepper.

Place the stuffed bell peppers in a baking dish and pour tomato sauce over them.

If desired, sprinkle vegan cheese on top.

Bake the dish for twenty-five to thirty minutes with the foil covering it.

Remove the foil and bake for an additional 10 minutes or until the peppers are tender.

Serve hot.

Cooking Time: 40 minutes

Total Making Time: 55 minutes

Serving Size: 4 servings

Nutrition Value (per serving):

Calories: 350

Protein: 12g

Fat: 7g

Carbohydrates: 62g

Fiber: 10g

Zucchini Noodles with Pesto:

Ingredients:

4 medium zucchinis, spiralized

1 cup cherry tomatoes, halved

1/2 cup black olives, sliced

1/4 cup pine nuts

1 cup fresh basil leaves

1/2 cup nutritional yeast

2 cloves garlic

1/2 cup extra-virgin olive oil

Salt and pepper to taste

Vegan Parmesan cheese for garnish (optional)

Preparation Method:

In a blender or food processor, combine basil, nutritional yeast, garlic, pine nuts, and olive oil. Blend until smooth.

In a large pan, sauté zucchini noodles until just tender.

Add cherry tomatoes and black olives to the pan, cooking for an additional 2-3 minutes.

Toss the zucchini noodles with pesto sauce until well coated.

Season with salt and pepper to taste.

Garnish with vegan Parmesan cheese if desired.

Serve immediately.

Cooking Time: 10 minutes

Total Making Time: 20 minutes

Serving Size: 2 servings

Nutrition Value (per serving):

Calories: 320

Protein: 8g

Fat: 28g

Carbohydrates: 12g

Fiber: 5g

Spaghetti Squash Primavera:

Ingredients:

1 medium spaghetti squash

1 cup cherry tomatoes, halved

1 cup broccoli florets

1 cup bell peppers, sliced

1/2 cup carrots, julienned

2 cloves garlic, minced

1/4 cup fresh basil, chopped

2 tablespoons olive oil

Salt and pepper to taste

Vegan Parmesan cheese for garnish (optional)

Preparation Method:

Preheat the oven to 400°F (200°C).

Cut the spaghetti squash in half lengthwise, scoop out the seeds, and place it cut-side down on a baking sheet.

Squash should be baked for 40 to 45 minutes, or until soft.

In a large pan, sauté garlic in olive oil until fragrant.

Add cherry tomatoes, broccoli, bell peppers, and carrots. Cook until vegetables are tender-crisp.

Use a fork to scrape the spaghetti squash strands into the pan with the vegetables.

Toss everything together until well combined.

Season with salt and pepper, garnish with fresh basil, and top with vegan Parmesan if desired.

Serve warm.

Cooking Time: 45 minutes

Total Making Time: 1 hour

Serving Size: 3 servings

Nutrition Value (per serving):

Calories: 220

Protein: 5g

Fat: 12g

Carbohydrates: 28g

Fiber: 7g

Lentil and Vegetable Curry:

Ingredients:

1 cup dry green or brown lentils, rinsed

1 large onion, diced

3 cloves garlic, minced

1 tablespoon ginger, grated

1 can (14 oz) diced tomatoes

1 can (14 oz) coconut milk

2 cups mixed vegetables (e.g., carrots, peas, bell peppers)

2 tablespoons curry powder

1 teaspoon cumin

1 teaspoon turmeric

Salt and pepper to taste

Fresh cilantro for garnish

Preparation Method:

In a large pot, sauté onions, garlic, and ginger until softened.

Add lentils, diced tomatoes, coconut milk, mixed vegetables, curry powder, cumin, turmeric, salt, and pepper.

Bring to a boil, then reduce heat and simmer until lentils are cooked and vegetables are tender.

Adjust seasoning to taste.

Garnish with fresh cilantro.

Serve over rice or quinoa.

Cooking Time: 30 minutes

Total Making Time: 45 minutes

Serving Size: 4 servings

Nutrition Value (per serving):

Calories: 380

Protein: 18g

Fat: 15g

Carbohydrates: 48g

Fiber: 15g

Vegan Sushi Bowl:

Ingredients:

2 cups sushi rice, cooked

1 cup tofu, cubed and marinated

1 cucumber, julienned

1 avocado, sliced

1 cup carrots, julienned

1/4 cup pickled ginger

1/4 cup soy sauce

1 tablespoon rice vinegar

1 tablespoon sesame oil

Sesame seeds for garnish

Nori strips for garnish

Preparation Method:

In a bowl, mix cooked sushi rice with rice vinegar and sesame oil.

Divide the rice among serving bowls.

Top with marinated tofu, cucumber, avocado, carrots, and pickled ginger.

Drizzle with soy sauce.

Garnish with sesame seeds and nori strips.

Serve and enjoy.

Cooking Time: 20 minutes

Total Making Time: 30 minutes

Serving Size: 2 servings

Nutrition Value (per serving):

Calories: 450

Protein: 15g

Fat: 12g

Carbohydrates: 70g

Fiber: 5g

Snacks recipes

Almond Butter and Banana Slices:

Ingredients:

Ripe bananas

Almond butter

Preparation Method:

Peel and slice the bananas.

Spread a layer of almond butter on each banana slice.

Instructions:

Arrange the almond butter-topped banana slices on a serving plate.

Cooking Time: None

Total Making Time: 5 minutes

Serving Size: 2

Nutrition Value (per serving):

Calories: 150

Protein: 3g

Fat: 8g

Carbohydrates: 18g

Fiber: 4g

Sugar: 8g

Carrot Sticks with Hummus:

Ingredients:

Carrot sticks

Hummus

Preparation Method:

Wash and peel the carrots.

Cut the carrots into stick shapes.

Serve with hummus for dipping.

Instructions:

Arrange the carrot sticks around a bowl of hummus.

Cooking Time: None

Total Making Time: 10 minutes

Serving Size: 4

Nutrition Value (per serving):

Calories: 80

Protein: 2g

Fat: 4g

Carbohydrates: 10g

Fiber: 3g

Sugar: 3g

Mixed Berry Parfait:

Ingredients:

Mixed berries (strawberries, blueberries, raspberries)

Dairy-free yogurt

Granola

Preparation Method:

Wash and prepare the berries.

In a glass or bowl, layer berries, yogurt, and granola.

Instructions:

Continue layering until the entire container is filled. Top with a few whole berries.

Cooking Time: None

Total Making Time: 15 minutes

Serving Size: 1

Nutrition Value (per serving):

Calories: 250

Protein: 6g

Fat: 8g

Carbohydrates: 40g

Fiber: 7g

Sugar: 15g

Kale Chips:

Ingredients:

Fresh kale leaves

Olive oil

Sea salt

Preparation Method:

Preheat the oven to 350°F (175°C).

Wash and dry the kale leaves. Take off the stems and shred into little pieces.

Toss the kale with olive oil and a pinch of sea salt.

Arrange the kale in a single layer on a baking pan.

Bake for 10-15 minutes until crisp.

Instructions:

Allow kale chips to cool before serving.

Cooking Time: 15 minutes

Total Making Time: 20 minutes

Serving Size: 2

Nutrition Value (per serving):

Calories: 80

Protein: 3g

Fat: 4g

Carbohydrates: 10g

Fiber: 3g

Sugar: 1g

Energy Bites:

Ingredients:

Dates

Almonds

Chia seeds

Cocoa powder

Preparation Method:

Dates and almonds should be processed in a food processor until a sticky mixture forms.

Add chia seeds and cocoa powder. Blend until well combined.

Roll the mixture into bite-sized balls.

Instructions:

Refrigerate energy bites for at least 30 minutes before serving.

Cooking Time: None

Total Making Time: 20 minutes

Serving Size: 8

Nutrition Value (per serving):

Calories: 100

Protein: 3g

Fat: 5g

Carbohydrates: 15g

Fiber: 4g

Sugar: 9g

Roasted Chickpeas:

Ingredients:

Canned chickpeas

Olive oil

Paprika

Cumin

Sea salt

Preparation Method:

Preheat the oven to 400°F (200°C).

Rinse and drain chickpeas, then pat dry.

Toss chickpeas with olive oil, paprika, cumin, and sea salt.

Spread chickpeas on a baking sheet in a single layer.

Roast for 20-25 minutes until crispy.

Instructions:

Let roasted chickpeas cool before serving.

Cooking Time: 25 minutes

Total Making Time: 30 minutes

Serving Size: 4

Nutrition Value (per serving):

Calories: 120

Protein: 4g

Fat: 2g

Carbohydrates: 20g

Fiber: 4g

Sugar: 4g

Veggie Sticks with Guacamole:

Ingredients:

Assorted vegetable sticks (carrots, cucumber, bell peppers)

Guacamole

Preparation Method:

Wash and cut vegetables into sticks.

Prepare or buy guacamole.

Instructions:

Arrange vegetable sticks around a bowl of guacamole.

Cooking Time: None

Total Making Time: 10 minutes

Serving Size: 4

Nutrition Value (per serving):

Calories: 90

Protein: 2g

Fat: 7g

Carbohydrates: 8g

Fiber: 4g

Sugar: 2g

Homemade Trail Mix:

Ingredients:

Mixed nuts (almonds, walnuts, cashews)

Dried fruits (raisins, cranberries)

Dark chocolate chips

Pumpkin seeds

Preparation Method:

Mix all ingredients in a bowl.

Instructions:

Store the trail mix in an airtight container.

Cooking Time: None

Total Making Time: 5 minutes

Serving Size: 6

Nutrition Value (per serving):

Calories: 150

Protein: 5g

Fat: 10g

Carbohydrates: 15g

Fiber: 3g

Sugar: 8g

Stuffed Dates:

Ingredients:

Dates

Almond butter

Chopped nuts

Preparation Method:

Slice dates and remove pits.

Fill each date with a small amount of almond butter.

Top with chopped nuts.

Instructions:

Serve stuffed dates immediately.

Cooking Time: None

Total Making Time: 10 minutes

Serving Size: 4

Nutrition Value (per serving):

Calories: 120

Protein: 2g

Fat: 5g

Carbohydrates: 20g

Fiber: 3g

Sugar: 15g

Edamame Pods:

Ingredients:

Edamame pods (frozen or fresh)

Sea salt

Preparation Method:

Boil or steam edamame pods until tender.

Sprinkle with sea salt.

Instructions:

Serve edamame pods in a bowl.

Cooking Time: 5 minutes

Total Making Time: 10 minutes

Serving Size: 2

Nutrition Value (per serving):

Calories: 100

Protein: 9g

Fat: 4g

Carbohydrates: 8g

Fiber: 4g

Sugar: 2g

Dessert recipes

Coconut Mango Sorbet:

Ingredients:

3 cups frozen mango chunks

1 can (14 ounces) coconut milk

1/4 cup maple syrup

1 tablespoon lime juice

Preparation Method:

In a blender, combine frozen mango chunks, coconut milk, maple syrup, and lime juice.

Blend until smooth.

Instructions:

Serve immediately for a soft sorbet or freeze for a firmer texture.

Garnish with fresh mint or shredded coconut.

Cooking Time: None (requires freezing time)

Total Making Time: 10 minutes

Serving Size: 4

Nutrition Value (per serving):

Calories: 220

Fat: 12g

Carbohydrates: 30g

Fiber: 3g

Protein: 2g

Vegan Berry Tart:

Ingredients:

1 pre-made vegan pie crust

1 cup dairy-free cream cheese

1/4 cup maple syrup

1 teaspoon vanilla extract

Assorted fresh berries for topping

Preparation Method:

In a bowl, whisk together dairy-free cream cheese, maple syrup, and vanilla extract until smooth.

Spread the mixture evenly over the pre-made pie crust.

Instructions:

Arrange fresh berries on top.

Before serving, place in the fridge for at least two hours.

Cooking Time: None (requires refrigeration time)

Total Making Time: 15 minutes

Serving Size: 8

Nutrition Value (per serving):

Calories: 180

Fat: 10g

Carbohydrates: 20g

Fiber: 2g

Protein: 2g

Chia Seed Pudding Parfait:

Ingredients:

1/2 cup chia seeds

2 cups almond milk

2 tablespoons maple syrup

1 teaspoon vanilla extract

Granola and fresh fruit for layering

Preparation Method:

In a bowl, mix chia seeds, almond milk, maple syrup, and vanilla extract.

Stir well and refrigerate overnight.

Instructions:

In serving glasses, layer the chia pudding with granola and fresh fruit.

Repeat the layers and top with additional fruit.

Cooking Time: Overnight (for chia pudding to set)

Total Making Time: 10 minutes (plus overnight refrigeration)

Serving Size: 4

Nutrition Value (per serving):

Calories: 180

Fat: 8g

Carbohydrates: 25g

Fiber: 8g

Protein: 5g

Frozen Banana Ice Cream:

Ingredients:

4 ripe bananas (sliced and frozen)

1/4 cup almond milk

1 teaspoon vanilla extract

Toppings of choice (nuts, chocolate chips, fruit)

Preparation Method:

Place frozen banana slices, almond milk, and vanilla extract in a blender.

Blend until smooth and creamy.

Instructions:

Transfer to a container and freeze for at least 2 hours for a firmer texture.

Scoop into bowls and add toppings of your choice.

Cooking Time: None (requires freezing time)

Total Making Time: 10 minutes (plus freezing time)

Serving Size: 4

Nutrition Value (per serving):

Calories: 120

Fat: 1g

Carbohydrates: 30g

Fiber: 3g

Protein: 1g

Pineapple Coconut Nice Cream:

Ingredients:

2 cups frozen pineapple chunks

1 can (14 ounces) coconut milk (full fat)

Two teaspoons of maple syrup (more sweetener optional)

1 teaspoon vanilla extract

Preparation Method:

Place the frozen pineapple chunks, coconut milk, maple syrup (if using), and vanilla extract in a blender.

Scrape down the sides as necessary, and blend until creamy and smooth.

Instructions:

Serve immediately as soft-serve or transfer to a container and freeze for a firmer texture.

Garnish with shredded coconut or fresh pineapple if desired.

Cooking Time: None (requires freezing time)

Total Making Time: 10 minutes

Serving Size: 4

Nutrition Value (per serving):

Calories: 180

Fat: 15g

Carbohydrates: 10g

Fiber: 2g

Protein: 1g

Berry Chia Seed Jam:

Ingredients:

2 cups mixed berries (strawberries, blueberries, raspberries)

2 tablespoons chia seeds

2 tablespoons maple syrup

1 tablespoon lemon juice

Preparation Method:

In a saucepan, combine the berries, chia seeds, maple syrup, and lemon juice.

Mash the berries with a fork and simmer on low heat until the mixture thickens.

Instructions:

Allow the jam to cool, and transfer it to a jar. Refrigerate until ready to use.

Spread on toast, yogurt, or use as a topping for desserts.

Cooking Time: 15 minutes

Total Making Time: 30 minutes

Serving Size: 8

Nutrition Value (per serving):

Calories: 50

Fat: 1g

Carbohydrates: 10g

Fiber: 3g

Protein: 1g

Almond Joy Energy Balls:

Ingredients:

1 cup almonds (raw, unsalted)

1 cup shredded coconut

1/2 cup dates (pitted)

2 tablespoons cocoa powder

1 tablespoon coconut oil

A pinch of sea salt

Preparation Method:

In a food processor, blend almonds until finely ground.

Add shredded coconut, dates, cocoa powder, coconut oil, and sea salt. Blend until the mixture sticks together.

Instructions:

Refrigerate for a minimum of half an hour after rolling the mixture into little balls.

Refrigerate and store in an airtight container.

Cooking Time: None (requires refrigeration time)

Total Making Time: 15 minutes

Serving Size: 12

Nutrition Value (per serving):

Calories: 120

Fat: 9g

Carbohydrates: 8g

Fiber: 3g

Protein: 3g

Banana Walnut Bread:

Ingredients:

3 ripe bananas (mashed)

1/3 cup coconut oil (melted)

1/2 cup maple syrup

1 teaspoon vanilla extract

2 cups whole wheat flour

1 teaspoon baking soda

1/2 teaspoon salt

1/2 cup chopped walnuts

Preparation Method:

Preheat the oven to 350°F (175°C). Grease a loaf pan.

In a large bowl, combine mashed bananas, melted coconut oil, maple syrup, and vanilla extract.

Mix the baking soda, salt, and flour in a separate basin. Add to the wet ingredients and mix until just combined.

Fold in chopped walnuts.

Instructions:

After filling the loaf pan, level the top of the batter.

When a toothpick put into the center comes out clean, bake for 60 to 65 minutes.

After letting the bread cool in the pan for ten minutes, move it to a wire rack to finish cooling.

Cooking Time: 60-65 minutes

Total Making Time: 1 hour, 30 minutes

Serving Size: 10

Nutrition Value (per serving):

Calories: 220

Fat: 10g

Carbohydrates: 30g

Fiber: 4g

Protein: 4g

Mango Coconut Rice Pudding:

Ingredients:

1 cup arborio rice

1 can (14 ounces) coconut milk

2 cups almond milk

1/2 cup maple syrup

1 teaspoon vanilla extract

1 cup mango (diced)

Shredded coconut for garnish

Preparation Method:

In a saucepan, combine arborio rice, coconut milk, almond milk, and maple syrup.

Bring to a simmer and cook, stirring occasionally, until the rice is cooked and the mixture has thickened.

Stir in vanilla extract and diced mango.

Instructions:

Serve warm or chilled, garnished with shredded coconut.

Cooking Time: 30 minutes

Total Making Time: 45 minutes

Serving Size: 6

Nutrition Value (per serving):

Calories: 350

Fat: 12g

Carbohydrates: 55g

Fiber: 2g

Protein: 4g

Avocado Chocolate Mousse:

Ingredients:

2 ripe avocados

1/4 cup cocoa powder

1/4 cup maple syrup

1 teaspoon vanilla extract

A pinch of salt

1/4 cup almond milk (as needed for consistency)

Preparation Method:

Once the avocados are scooped out, add them to a blender.

Mix in vanilla essence, maple syrup, cocoa powder, and a small amount of salt.

Blend until smooth, adding almond milk as needed for a creamy consistency.

Instructions:

Before serving, place in the fridge for at least two hours.

Garnish with fresh berries or nuts if desired.

Cooking Time: None (requires refrigeration time)

Total Making Time: 10 minutes

Serving Size: 4

Nutrition Value (per serving):

Calories: 180

Fat: 12g

Carbohydrates: 20g

Fiber: 6g

Protein: 3g

Healthy fruit to include

Watermelon:

Hydration Benefit: Watermelon is composed of over 90% water, providing excellent hydration for the skin.

Hygiene: Wash the outer rind thoroughly before cutting.

Eating Time: Ideal for hot summer days or as a refreshing snack.

Portion: One cup of diced watermelon.

Nutrition Value:

Calories: 46

Water Content: About 92%

Vitamins: A, C

Tips: Include watermelon cubes in salads or blend into a hydrating smoothie.

Cucumber:

Hydration Benefit: Cucumbers are rich in water, promoting skin hydration.

Hygiene: Wash and peel if not organic, or scrub thoroughly.

Eating Time: Anytime, as a snack or added to salads.

Portion: One medium cucumber.

Nutrition Value:

Calories: 45

Water Content: About 95%

Vitamins: K, C

Tips: Slice cucumbers for a light and hydrating snack or use in infused water.

Strawberries:

Hydration Benefit: Strawberries contain water and antioxidants for skin health.

Hygiene: Rinse under cold water before consuming.

Eating Time: Breakfast, snacks, or dessert.

Portion: One cup of whole strawberries.

Nutrition Value:

Calories: 49

Water Content: About 91%

Vitamins: C, manganese

Tips: Add strawberries to yogurt or enjoy them as a standalone snack.

Pineapple:

Hydration Benefit: Pineapple offers hydration and contains enzymes for digestion.

Hygiene: Peel and cut into slices or chunks.

Eating Time: Mid-morning or as a tropical dessert.

Portion: One cup of pineapple chunks.

Nutrition Value:

Calories: 82

Water Content: About 86%

Vitamins: C, B6

Tips: Mix pineapple into fruit salads or make a refreshing pineapple smoothie.

Oranges:

Hydration Benefit: Oranges are juicy and high in vitamin C, promoting skin elasticity.

Hygiene: Peel and separate into segments.

Eating Time: Morning or as a snack.

Portion: One medium-sized orange.

Nutrition Value:

Calories: 62

Water Content: About 87%

Vitamins: C, A

Tips: Make fresh orange juice or add orange slices to salads.

Grapefruit:

Hydration Benefit: Grapefruit provides hydration and antioxidants.

Hygiene: Cut and peel the sections or slice into wedges.

Eating Time: Breakfast or as a tangy snack.

Portion: Half a grapefruit.

Nutrition Value:

Calories: 52

Water Content: About 88%

Vitamins: C, A

Tips: Sprinkle a little honey on top for added sweetness.

Tips for Radiant Skin:

Stay Hydrated: In addition to consuming hydrating fruits, drink plenty of water throughout the day.

Balanced Diet: Include a variety of fruits, vegetables, and whole foods for overall skin health.

Limit Sugary Intake: While fruits are healthy, moderation is key, especially for fruits higher in natural sugars.

Protect Your Skin: To shield your skin from damaging UV radiation, apply sunscreen.

Practice Good Skincare: Establish a regular skincare routine to cleanse, moisturize, and protect your skin.

Remember, radiant skin is often a reflection of overall health, so adopting a holistic approach to your lifestyle and diet can have a positive impact on your skin's appearance and health.

CHAPTER 5:
TRANSITIONING FROM THE KITCHEN TO THE VANITY

DIY Beauty Treatments: Harnessing the Power of Plants

In the quest for radiant and healthy skin, harnessing the power of plants through DIY beauty treatments has become a popular and effective approach. These natural remedies not only pamper your skin but also provide it with the nourishment it needs to glow from the inside out. From homemade masks to natural cleansers and plant-powered moisturizers, here's a comprehensive guide to elevating your skincare routine with botanical wonders.

Homemade Masks for Radiant Skin:

Avocado and Honey Mask:

Ingredients: Mashed avocado, raw honey.

Benefits: Avocado nourishes with essential fatty acids, while honey adds natural antibacterial properties and hydration.

Turmeric and Yogurt Mask:

Ingredients: Turmeric powder, plain yogurt.

Benefits: Turmeric's anti-inflammatory properties combined with yogurt's lactic acid help brighten and soothe the skin.

Oatmeal and Banana Mask:

Ingredients: Ground oatmeal, mashed banana.

Benefits: Oatmeal exfoliates gently, and banana provides vitamins for a soft and supple complexion.

Strawberry and Lemon Mask:

Ingredients: Mashed strawberries, fresh lemon juice.

Benefits: Strawberries offer antioxidants, while lemon brightens and tones the skin.

Natural Cleansers and Toners:

Cucumber and Aloe Vera Cleanser:

Ingredients: Blended cucumber, aloe vera gel.

Benefits: Cucumber soothes, and aloe vera cleanses, leaving your skin refreshed and hydrated.

Green Tea Toner:

Ingredients: Brewed green tea, witch hazel.

Benefits: Green tea is rich in antioxidants, and witch hazel helps tone and tighten the skin.

Rosewater and Glycerin Toner:

Ingredients: Rosewater, glycerin.

Benefits: Rosewater has anti-inflammatory properties, while glycerin moisturizes and maintains skin elasticity.

Apple Cider Vinegar Cleanser:

Ingredients: Diluted apple cider vinegar, water.

Benefits: Balances the skin's pH, unclogs pores, and has antibacterial properties.

Plant-Powered Moisturizers:

Coconut Oil and Lavender Moisturizer:

Ingredients: Coconut oil, lavender essential oil.

Benefits: Coconut oil provides deep hydration, and lavender oil soothes and calms the skin.

Shea Butter and Jojoba Oil Moisturizer:

Ingredients: Shea butter, jojoba oil.

Benefits: Shea butter is rich in vitamins, and jojoba oil mimics the skin's natural oils, providing intense hydration.

Aloe Vera Gel and Almond Oil Moisturizer:

Ingredients: Aloe Vera gel, almond oil.

Benefits: Aloe Vera soothes and hydrates, while almond oil nourishes and promotes a radiant complexion.

Argan Oil and Rosehip Seed Oil Moisturizer:

Ingredients: Argan oil, rosehip seed oil.

Benefits: Argan oil is rich in antioxidants, and rosehip seed oil helps with cell regeneration and collagen production.

Embracing these DIY beauty treatments allows you to indulge in the goodness of plants while tailoring your skincare routine to your unique needs. Experiment with these natural ingredients to discover the perfect blend that will leave your skin looking and feeling its best. Remember to patch-test new ingredients and enjoy the journey to naturally radiant skin.

Chapter 6: Beyond the Plate

The Comprehensive Guide to Radiant Skin through a Holistic Approach

Using a holistic strategy that takes into account many parts of your lifestyle is necessary to get glowing skin, which goes beyond skincare products. This thorough book examines how stress reduction, physical activity, and restful sleep are all related to bright, glowing skin.

Stress Reduction for Clear Skin: Stress is a typical issue that can have a big impact on the condition of your skin. Prolonged stress causes the production of cortisol, a hormone that can cause inflammation and skin problems in excess. Using stress-reduction strategies is crucial to keeping skin bright and clean.

Stress levels have been demonstrated to decrease with mindfulness meditation practice. Locate a peaceful area, pay attention to your breathing, and release tension.

Yoga and Relaxation Techniques: Doing yoga or other relaxation techniques can help release stress and encourage serenity, which will improve the appearance of your skin.

Healthy Coping strategies: To effectively manage stress, cultivate healthy coping strategies like writing, chatting to friends, or engaging in a hobby.

Exercise's Effect on Skin Health: Exercising on a regular basis helps your skin look radiant while also improving your general health. Increased blood circulation from exercise helps maintain and nourish healthy skin cells.

Cardiovascular Exercise: Exercises that stimulate blood flow, such as riding, dancing, or jogging, help the skin receive nutrients and oxygen.

Strength Training: Strength training increases muscular mass, which improves the firmness and suppleness of the skin.

Post-Workout Skincare: To avoid clogged pores, wash your skin right away after working out to get rid of sweat and pollutants.

The Value of Restful Sleep: A comprehensive strategy for glowing skin must include getting enough sleep. The body repairs and regenerates itself when you sleep, and this includes skin cell renewal. Sleep deprivation can worsen skin health by raising stress hormones and inflammatory markers.

Establish a Sleep pattern: To control your body's internal clock, establish a regular sleep pattern.

Establish a Calm Environment: Make sure your bedroom is quiet, well-lit, and at a temperature that is pleasant for sleeping in.

Limit Your Screen Time Before Bed: The hormone melatonin, which is necessary for sleep, can be disrupted by spending time in front of a screen before bed.

Achieving a balanced lifestyle and skincare regimen is essential to holistically achieving glowing skin. Clear, radiant skin that represents your entire health is built on a foundation of stress management, regular exercise, and restful sleep. Recall that maintaining long-term skin health and brightness requires persistence in these procedures.

CONCLUSION

In conclusion, embracing a vegan diet for radiant skin is not just a dietary choice; it's a lifestyle that nurtures overall well-being. Throughout this exploration of plant-based nutrition, we've uncovered the profound connection between what we consume and the luminosity of our skin. From understanding the link between diet and skin health to delving into essential nutrients, antioxidants, and the beauty of plant-based foods, each chapter has unveiled the transformative power of a vegan lifestyle.

By choosing plant-powered meals, individuals can witness a positive metamorphosis in their skin's radiance. The array of fruits, vegetables, nuts, and grains not only provides essential vitamins and minerals but also offers hydration, nourishment, and protection against oxidative stress. Homemade recipes, from vibrant smoothie bowls to nutrient-packed salads, serve as a testament to the delicious possibilities within the realm of vegan culinary creativity.

However, radiant skin transcends the realm of mere physical appearance; it reflects a harmonious interplay of internal health and external care. Thus, our journey has also explored the significance of stress management, regular exercise, and restful sleep as integral components of a holistic approach to skin wellness.

As you embark on this journey toward a vegan diet for radiant skin, let it be a celebration of nourishment, compassion, and self-love. By choosing the vibrant colors of nature over processed alternatives, you not only enhance your skin's glow but also contribute to a sustainable and compassionate lifestyle. Remember, the beauty of radiant skin lies not just in its visual appeal but in the vitality it mirrors from within.

So, to every reader considering or already on this path, I offer a special motivation: embrace this journey with joy and curiosity. Explore the rich tapestry of plant-based foods, savor the flavors, and revel in the positive changes unfolding within you. Let your choice be a commitment not just to your skin but to the planet and all its inhabitants. As you nourish your body with the goodness of the earth, may your radiant skin be a reflection of the radiant soul embracing a lifestyle that is as beautiful as it is compassionate. Cheers to the journey of vibrant well-being, one plant-based bite at a time!